Glow Up Your Life!

Glow Up Your Life!

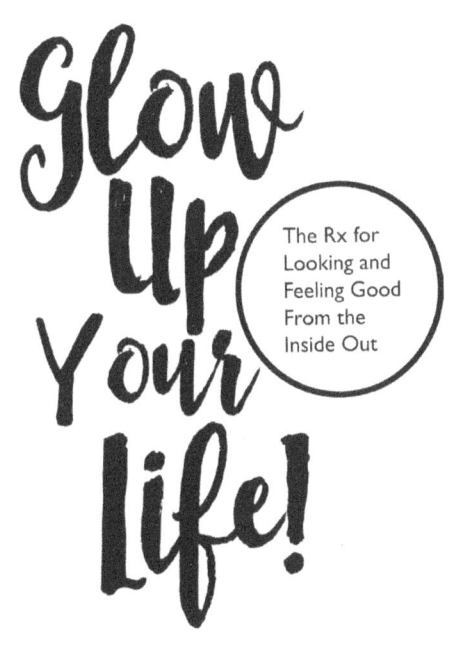

The Rx for Looking and Feeling Good From the Inside Out

Kristamarie F. Collman, MD

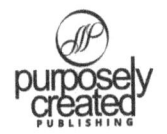

purposely created
PUBLISHING

GLOW UP YOUR LIFE!

Published by Purposely Created Publishing Group™

Copyright © 2019 Kristamarie F. Collman

All rights reserved.

No part of this book may be reproduced, distributed or transmitted in any form by any means, graphic, electronic, or mechanical, including photocopy, recording, taping, or by any information storage or retrieval system, without permission in writing from the publisher, except in the case of reprints in the context of reviews, quotes, or references.
Printed in the United States of America

ISBN: 978-1-64484-900-2

Special discounts are available on bulk quantity purchases by book clubs, associations and special interest groups. For details email: sales@publishyourgift.com or call (888) 949-6228.

For information log on to www.PublishYourGift.com

Table of Contents

Acknowledgments vii

Introduction 1

Part One: Inner Glow Up

Chapter 1: Loving What You See in the Mirror 7

Chapter 2: Developing Your Own Mantra 13

Chapter 3: Glowing Up with Gratitude 17

Chapter 4: Eat to Glow 23

Chapter 5: Stress Less, Glow More 31

Part Two: Outer Glow Up

Chapter 6: Cleaning Out the Closet 41

Chapter 7: Shopping on a Budget 49

Chapter 8: Dressing for Your Body Type 55

Chapter 9: Travel Wear 61

Chapter 10: Dressing for the Werk Out 67

Chapter 11: Choosing Accessories for You 75

Chapter 12: Appearance in the Professional Space 87

BONUS: Style on Point, How About Your
Professional Skills? 95

BONUS: Don't Let Your Light Burn Out 103

Thank You 111

About the Author 113

Acknowledgments

I wrote this book for my sisters who are all beautiful in their own skin and have so much to share with the world. For the beautiful sister who struggles with making sure she not only looks good but feels good. The ones who have moments of self-doubt and often question what they see in the mirror. The wife, fiancé, mom, woman in school juggling multiple jobs, CEO, doctor, lawyer, auntie, and bestie who excels in everything she sets forth to do, yet still feels like she has so much to say to a world that is not listening. For the beauty trying to live up to society's definition of beautiful, I get it and I feel you. I am you.

I thank God for that moment in life where I was not mentally, physically, or spiritually healthy. For the breaking point early in my modeling career, which shattered my self-confidence and made me feel completely worthless during a photo shoot. I had done such a great job at making everything look picture perfect that no one around me knew what was going on, but I knew I had to make some major changes in my life. My weight was fluctuating in an unhealthy manner, my self-assurance was at an all-time low, and I didn't even recognize the woman staring back at me when I looked in the mirror. This experience gave me the tenacity to control my health and realize that I had the power to define my own beauty and refuse to be held to anyone else's definition of what I should look like in order to be beautiful. And I want to share how you can discover this too!

Yours in Health and Style,

Dr. Kristamarie

Introduction

Let me share my real story with you: My parents immigrated here from Jamaica, and with no doctors in my family, becoming a physician was only a dream. But growing up, I worked very hard to make that dream a reality. I was raised in the suburbs of New Jersey and graduated with honors from Rutgers, The State University of New Jersey, with a degree in public health and a minor in biology. I was later gifted acceptance and a partial scholarship to attend New York Medical College. After earning my medical degree, I completed my residency in family medicine, where I was nominated and chosen to serve as chief resident. It was also during my residency where I met H, who's now my fiancé.

To everyone looking in, I appeared to have the perfect life—on the path to a successful career and happily in love with everything altogether. But I have experienced my fair share of downsides.

Let me take you back to my college years.

I juggled numerous jobs and enjoyed modeling on the side. One Thursday evening, I was in Manhattan on set for a photoshoot. I'd finished taking my round of pictures and thought to myself, I nailed it! After all, I had been preparing for this shoot for weeks and had been meticulously watching my diet. After we finished taking my pictures, the photographer called me over to review the photos. He scrolled through each one, shaking his head no, nope, no. I watched him as he took his eraser and slimmed down my waist. Then my hips. Then my thighs. My self-confidence was completely shattered to an all-time low. This experience left me feeling insecure with negative thoughts brewing about my body and feeling like I was not good enough. Friends and family close to me noticed a change in my appearance and attitude. Not to mention I had compromised my health by developing unhealthy habits like smoking and skipping meals to maintain my appearance. My mood began to change, as I gave up on taking care of my looks. When I looked in the mirror, I did not recognize the woman staring back at me.

After this experience, I said by "bye bye" to my model dreams and continued on the journey in medicine. I made the decision that I was going to implement positive lifestyle changes to live as happy and healthy as I could. One by one, I started making small changes that helped me on the path to success. However, something deep down within me knew that being a doctor was not the end all be all. I knew that I had a higher purpose.

As I reflected on my journey to "Dr. Kristamarie," I remembered my college self and how I never want women to feel the way I did when that photographer looked at me in disapproval. That is why I have committed myself to helping women feel great about themselves—to feel beautiful, look beautiful, and accomplish their dreams.

This experience fueled my desire to serve as a source for career inspiration while helping women feel healthy, confident and bold through adapting healthy lifestyle habits and improving their style savvy. The clothes we wear have an uncanny ability to help us feel beautiful and confident, whether we notice it or not. When this is paired with healthy lifestyle choices, it's a recipe for success! My love for style, fashion, and healthy living inspired me to help women such as yourself rediscover your beauty, feel confident in your skin, and find that inner boss so that you can share your message with the world too. What exactly does glow up mean? It's certainly more than just the alteration of a person's outer appearance. I see a "glow up" as a comprehensive transformation where an individual is healthy, feels fabulous on the inside and out, all while conquering their goals. Remember, you don't have to keep looking beyond yourself for a model of "goals." You are goals and I'm here to help you take shape.

Part One

Inner Glow Up

Chapter 1
Loving What You See in the Mirror

―◆―

"Beauty begins the moment you decide to be yourself."
– Diane V. Furstenberg

Don't give a d@mn what others think. People will always have an opinion, whether you ask them for it or not. I found myself always trying to live up to everyone else's expectations, and THIS IS IMPOSSIBLE. To be honest, people don't care about us as much as we think they do. Once we get over the fear of what others are thinking, we gain a special sense of freedom, our happiness increases, and we can love our true self.

SHIFTING FOCUS

I used to focus exclusively on how I looked on the outside and would ruminate over particular areas of my body. The more we dwell on a particular feature of our body, the more of an issue it becomes. But what if we focused on how we felt on the INSIDE? Instead of focusing on how my body looked from the outside, I began thinking of all the wonderful strengths my body had from the inside. And I want you to do the same.

LISTENING TO YOUR BODY

Our body actually speaks to us. It tells us what it likes and how it feels by these feel-good brain chemicals called neurotransmitters. There are numerous ways to increase these feel-good hormones, from the foods we eat to the exercises we partake in. Our clothing, although not directly linked to feel-good hormones, can certainly evoke good feelings and emotions.

AVOID NEGATIVE SELF-TALK

Thoughts move through our brain through different pathways. The more negative thoughts we have, the stronger these pathways become. This often becomes a vicious cycle. Help your brain rewire itself with some kind thoughts and self-love.

KNOW THYSELF

Do you really know yourself? What are your strengths? Are you a people person? Which activities do you truly enjoy doing day in and day out? In order to accept myself, I had to understand who that woman staring at me was when I looked in the mirror. I had to stop trying to be so perfect because perfection is so hard to love (not to mention it's also boring)! Take some time to date yourself, enjoy your own company, and rediscover the things that make you beautiful!

Notes

Notes

Notes

Notes

Chapter 2
Developing Your Own Mantra

"Perseverance is failing 19 times and succeeding the 20th."

—Julie Andrews

A mantra is a positive thought or affirmation used to inspire you to be your best and support the way you want to live. As we are on the path to glowing up our life, there are experiences, which require us to focus our minds. A mantra serves as an additional source of encouragement for us to reach our goals. Yes, it's great to look at messages that others have shared, but it is not the same as something that comes from YOU.

I know you're asking, Dr. Kristamarie, why do we need a mantra? On life's journey, there will always be challenges and times where we are tested. There will be moments that seem as if nothing is going your way, where you experience self-doubt, consistently ruminate over decisions, or wonder if you are capable of achieving your goals. When there are so many distractions occurring around you, a mantra helps you gain clarity and serves as a source of motivation to move past these moments.

In medical school, which was one of the toughest times of my life, I used the mantra "I am strong and I can do this." I began to truly absorb this, and when I doubted my abilities, this mantra helped me stay strong and move forward. For us to truly experience a glow up, you have to be your biggest advocate.

Again, this will act as your personal slogan; it can be a quote or a powerful statement that you create yourself. There is no right or wrong mantra. Take a moment to sit quietly and think about what you would like your personal mantra to be. You can have multiple mantras, but you should focus on one at a time. Write it down on the next page and dedicate five minutes daily to repeating and truly believing your mantra.

Write Your Own Mantra

Chapter 3
Glowing Up with Gratitude

"Be thankful for what you have; you'll end up having more. If you concentrate on what you don't have, you will never, ever have enough."

– **Oprah**

When we show appreciation, our inner glow will shine so bright, others will start to take notice. When you show appreciation for whatever shows up, it changes your vibe and generates more great things to come your way.

It was just a few years ago that I started keeping a gratitude journal. Prior to this, I was so focused on my difficult path to becoming a doctor that I lost sight of being grateful for simply having a path to walk on. One of my coaches recommended that I begin a gratitude journal to remind me of the all the good things (no matter how small) occurring that I should be mindful and appreciative of. Once I began to feel gratitude for all of the events I encountered, including the opportunity to serve other women, I noticed a shift on the inside and out.

There have been numerous studies, which have found that people who wrote about their gratitude showed greater signs of emotional well-being.

You can start practicing an attitude of gratitude in small ways. Having a gratitude list doesn't have to consist of only huge moments that happen; it can simply be for having a cup of clean water to drink or the moment with a special friend. The trick is to be fully present in the moment of appreciation by noting why you are thankful. The act of writing down what you are grateful for is a great way to ensure all the details so that you don't forget it. The best part, however, is that by keeping a journal or notepad, you are able to refer to the journal or notepad anytime you are feeling low. Talk about an instant glow right there! There are tons to be grateful for, once we learn to look for it. Take a moment right now to jot down three things that you are grateful for.

Notes

Notes

Notes

Notes

Chapter 4
Eat to Glow

"You are what you eat. So don't be fast, cheap or fake."

– Unknown

Just as important as it is to dress right, it's equally important to make sure your health is on the right path. Nutrition and eating the right foods help us to feel good on the inside so that we can shine on the outside in our clothes. There is no other experience than feeling empowered and in control of your health. This is not a chapter on everything we need to know about food and nutrition (that has its own book), but I am touching on a few principles that can get (and keep) our health on the right track.

LOVE YOUR CARBS

Carbs are essential for the functioning of our bodies and giving our brain energy! What's important to keep in mind is to limit the bad carbs and have more of the good carbohydrates. Keep in mind I did not say eliminate all carbs. Items such as bagels, white potatoes, and white bread cause our blood sugar to spike, which is a huge red flag! When this happens, our risk for diseases such as diabetes and cardiovascular disease increases. Which carbs should we be eating more of? Think beans, whole grains, vegetables, and fruits. These are the carbs that have an abundance of vitamins, minerals, and other health-boosting nutrients.

EATING THOSE FRUITS AND VEGGIES

These are some of the best foods that we have in our arsenal for our health! For vegetables, the goal should be to consume 4-5 servings per day. For fruits, aim for 1-2 servings a day (though it may change if you have diabetes or are overweight). Colorful vegetables and fruits can help to protect and improve our health. The more colorful and brighter the color of the fruit or vegetable, the higher its nutritional power.

CHECK YOUR DRINK

It is also essential to make sure you are drinking the right beverages and that you are getting the right amount of water. Sugary drinks like sports drinks and soda have high amounts of calories and send our blood sugars through the roof, increasing the risk for weight gain. How does this happen? When our blood sugar peaks, it tells our body to store fat, not burn fat, and makes us hungrier. Options such as fruit-flavored water or teas are options. Also, when eating out, especially at restaurants, one of my tips for beverages is either water or wine. Red wine particularly has been associated with numerous health benefits and is a healthier option than mixed alcoholic drinks, which may be high in sugar.

Notes

Notes

Notes

Notes

Chapter 5
Stress Less, Glow More

"The day she let go of the things that were weighing her down, was the day she began to shine the brightest"

– Katrina Mayer

What exactly is stress? Through my knowledge and personal journey with stress, I see it as our body's reaction and energy released in response to any circumstance in order to survive. Stress causes the release of many different hormones inside our bodies, which can wreak havoc on our organs. The changes often lead to weight gain, increase our risk for diabetes and heart disease, cause hair loss, worsen acne, impact our sex lives, our ability sleep, our memory, and so much more. While stress can certainly cause negative changes on the inside of our bodies, stress can impact our ability to shine on the outside.

We know that stress is something we cannot avoid and it's becoming more common in today's modern world. However, not all stress is bad for us. Small doses of stress (what we experience when taking an important exam or during an interview) can keep us on our toes and improve our performance. The issue occurs when stress happens persistently over long periods of time. Stress can impact our emotional, mental and physical health. How can we reduce our stress levels, allowing our glow to shine? It's impossible for me to go into all the detail in this book, but I can state a few things below that have worked personally for me when dealing with stress:

- Learn to say no: Quite often, we can succumb to being "the yes person" and overcommitting ourselves to family, friends and work obligations. As busy women, we are often wearing so many different hats. The next time someone asks you to do something, and you don't want to or cannot, remember that "no" is a respectable answer as well.

- Laugh and smile: It has been said that laughter is the best medicine. I truly believe this. Sometimes, just cracking a smile or having a small laugh can improve your mood and lower your stress levels.

- Living an active life: Physical activity or exercise can be therapeutic for high stress levels! Not only can it help to treat stress, but it can help to prevent it as well! Your activity doesn't have to include spending hours in the gym. Studies have shown that small amounts of physical activity can have tremendous impact.

- Sip the tea: Literally! Take a moment, be it five minutes, to have a cup of warm tea. Use this moment to focus solely on yourself. I enjoy sipping herbal tea without caffeine, as caffeine can serve as a stimulant and worsen the feelings we may experience during stressful circumstances. Having a moment to yourself with a cup of tea or any other warm beverage can provide a stress relieving moment.

The art of stressing less is different for everyone. Once you learn how to manage stress in the best way possible for YOU, you will be able to glow like no one else!

Notes

Notes

Notes

Notes

Part Two

---◆---

Outer Glow Up

Chapter 6
Cleaning Out the Closet

Often it's what we hold onto that holds us back.

THE MENTAL AND PHYSICAL CLOSET

Cleaning out the closet is not just for spring; it can be done at any time. Additionally, we have to clean out two closets—first, our mental closet and second, our physical closet. When I had my breaking point, I had done such a good job at curating the perfect life, no one had any idea of the things I was going through. I had to come clean about my past and my truth so that I could help others! Sisters, this is the first step to cleaning out the mental closet—being genuine and forthright with your story, because you have a gift that someone else needs to hear. And if our physical closet is a mess, what does that say about other aspects of our lives? Getting in formation and having our bedroom closet in some type of order can provide clarity and allow us to focus on other more important areas of our lives.

First Step: Set aside time.

This can be a daunting task, so it will be important to set aside a few hours to go through every single item. If this still sounds like too much, you can divide and conquer. One day you can tackle tops, dresses or shoes the next day, and so forth. Make sure you set aside additional time for follow-up duties which may be needed after a closet haul (e.g. driving to donation stores or to the post office to mail goods and packages off).

Second Step: Ask These Six Questions

- Have I worn this in the past 12 months?
- Does it fit exactly how I want it to fit?
- Does it make me feel good and confident when I wear it?
- Is it currently in season?
- Do I have some sort of attachment or sentimental value to it?
- Is this a staple or basic?

If the answer is a solid no to any of the above, then remove the item(s) promptly from the closet and toss into one of four piles: Sell. Donate. Store. Trash.

Sell

This pile will be for items that you definitely don't wear. These items may be brand new (or slightly worn and are not damaged), and someone else may get some good use out of. It's a great way to easily make a small profit on your unused goods. You could consider traditional online stores such as eBay, but recently there has been an emergence of online social marketplaces that can be found with an easy Google search.

Donate

These are items that are still in good condition but are not sellable. However, someone may still benefit from its use. Some organizations may even pick them up from your home, depending on the location. In addition to organizations such as Goodwill, there are numerous not-for-profit organizations that would appreciate your donations. One of my favorite organizations accepts gently used professional clothing to help disadvantaged women who are entering or returning to the workplace. Take into account your values and goals, which can influence who you decide to donate items to.

Store

This pile will be for the items you still wear because they fit and give you good feels. You can decide to stores items in a separate closet if you have this or air-tight containers.

Be mindful of storage areas that may be exposed to weather (such as heat) because certain temperatures can affect the material of the clothing.

Trash

I'm not sure if this needs an explanation, but I'll give it anyway because it can be hard to let go of little things. These will be the items that you no longer want because they are stained, torn, or no longer in wearable condition. I will share that I like to keep items from my younger school days for nostalgia (like sports tees and shirts from social events). Instead of keeping an entire drawer full of tees, I had a quilt made out of the t-shirt squares for me to keep around.

MOVING FORWARD

Sometimes we have to let things go and give ourselves a fresh start ahead of us. There's no need to keep all five plaid shirts; consider getting rid of at least one or three of them. Trust me, you will not miss them.

Notes

Notes

Notes

Notes

Chapter 7
Shopping on a Budget

"Money talks, style doesn't have to."
—Unknown

My auntie used to say "Kris, even if what you're wearing costs $5, if you wear it confidently, it'll look like a million bucks." She was the original budgetista for buying clothes! Over the years, she taught me a few tips on securing the bags and saving coins when it comes to shopping:

KNOWING WHAT YOU ALREADY HAVE

Before you run out to go buy new clothes, check what's already in your closet! Sometimes there may be fashion gems tucked away that, once discovered, can turn into several outfits.

TIMING OF SHOPPING

Try shopping at the end of season to save those coins! For example, get a few summer clothes towards the beginning of fall season when the stores are trying to make space for fall gear. You will wait a little longer to wear it, but the money you will save will make it worth it.

FAVORITE PLACES TO SAVE ON STYLE

Brands such as Louis Vuitton, Chanel, and Gucci can really put a damper on a bank account, but you can score these brands and more at significantly discounted prices if you check out consignment stores. These are stores that sell secondhand clothing and accessories that are usually in great condition. I have also found items (some which have never been used) on sale. It really is like a gold mine! Stores such as TJ Maxx and Kohls (their motto: known for breaking hearts, not banks) are other stores to snag trendy items at a fraction of the cost.

ONLINE SHOPPING

Online shopping has become more popular over the past few years, especially since it is super convenient and you don't have to worry about long lines for the fitting room or to check out. You can find deals on sites such as Amazon and thredUP. However, shopping online can be a challenge as you have to learn which brands you like and also know your sizes. You also want to double check the return policy and make sure the company is flexible with returns and exchanges.

Notes

Notes

Notes

Notes

Chapter 8
Dressing for Your Body Type

"Style is a way to say who you are without having to speak."

—Rachel Zoe

What issa body type? Your body type is the outline of your structure as defined by our body parts. It is important to make sure the outfits we choose fit according to our proportions and sit beautifully along our figure. It's also important that pieces enhance and not take away from our silhouette.

NO MORE FRUIT (TO COMPARE US TO THAT IS)

When I used to open up fashion magazines, I would come across different body types compared to various pieces of fruits—banana, pear, apple. I'm not sure about you, but the last time I checked, I wasn't a piece of fruit. I am a beautiful human being. I also wondered what it meant if I didn't fit into one of the fruit categories? We all want to feel like we fit in somewhere, right?

STYLES FOR YOUR BODY SHAPE

The reality is, we are all shaped differently and that's what makes us beautiful. However, getting dressed when you know which pieces compliment your shape can make the process a little easier. For example, if you tend to gain weight in the midsection, consider more slim cut pants and tops with a waistline right below the bust. Avoid styles that draw attention to the middle like high rise pants. If you have narrow shoulders with a larger hip area, try items such as tapered A-line skirts (skirts that taper out gently from a narrow waist, making the shape of the capital letter A). If you have a straight up and down look, you may consider avoiding dresses that are tight all over. What's most important to remember though is if you are comfortable and confident, you will look great no matter what.

Notes

Notes

Notes

Notes

Chapter 9
Travel Wear

---◆---

"The secret of great style is to feel good in what you wear."

—Ines de La Fressange

DRESSING ON THE GO

Professional women are always getting ready to go somewhere. Whether it's on a business trip or a quick weekend away with the girls (or for some much needed alone time), it's important to know how to pack when you're ready to jet. The key is to have luggage with lots of compartments but that still meet requirements for carry-on size. Samsonite is one of my favorite brands, but there are many others available.

When flying, you want to travel in style but comfortable. You also want to be prepared for cooler temperatures as planes typically have the A/C high. So bringing a sweater or jacket is a must. If you are checking in luggage, you want to prepare an oversized tote with essentials (and include one spare outfit in case the checked bag gets lost).

PACKING AN OVERNIGHT BAG

Although it sounds simple, it may be helpful to keep a checklist of items needed nearby so that nothing is forgotten. I like to keep a running list of items such as my charger and certain pieces of jewelry as a list for reference. Consider also keeping a pre-prepped toiletry bag ready with the essentials needed. This is where you keep travel-sized items (e.g. toothpaste, facial cleanser, mouthwash, shampoos, etc.) handy so that when you have to leave, it's ready and you won't have forgotten your important nighttime face cream.

Notes

Notes

Notes

Notes

Chapter 10
Dressing for the Werk Out

We will feel even better in our clothes when we are keeping up with our physical health. Whether we are at the gym or outside, our clothing can have an impact on our exercise.

WERKING OUT CONFIDENTLY

Workout gear should certainly make you feel confident and strong! This is essential when heading to the gym or even performing an at-home workout. Our gear can motivate us to get our physical activity in and even finish the workout!

WERKING OUT IN STYLE

Finding cute workout gear can also be a motivating factor for working out. Tip here, you want it to be stylish AND functional. If you don't have time to go to the store to find outfits, you can consider workout gear subscription boxes where you receive 1-2 complete outfits for a discounted monthly price.

Breathable gear

You not only want to be in style when working out, but you want to make sure your gear is functional. Your particular activity can help determine which fabrics are best. Cotton, which is great for absorbing moisture, would be great for low sweat activities or yoga. For an intense workout, consider nylon based items—soft on the skin, breathable, and dries quickly. Brands such as Nike and Brooks create workout gear that can improve your sweat session.

Finding the right shoes

One of the most important items for the gym is our foot gear. Not wearing the right foot wear when working out can increase the risk for foot injury. The specific type of shoes will vary based on your workout or sport. From cross trainers to running shoes to tennis shoes, there is a shoe for almost every workout.

Support for the girls

Wearing a sports bra while working out is an important part of breast care and protection. Breasts are composed of lots of fatty tissue and special ligaments called Cooper's ligaments. Once these ligaments are stretched or broken down over time, the breasts will sag and there's no coming back from that. Sports bras help to support these ligaments. In some cases, if you exercise without a bra, this can increase the risk for breast or back pain. How do we choose the right bra? This will depend on a number of factors, including your cup size and activity level. Comfort is important, so you want to find light fabrics that absorb sweat and allow for lots of movement. It's always important to buy a good quality sports bra to help support your body, which, in turn, will improve your workouts.

Notes

Notes

Notes

Notes

Chapter 11
Choosing Accessories for You

---◆---

PART 1: JEWELRY ESSENTIALS

"I've always thought of accessories as the exclamation point of a woman's outfit."

—Michael K.

Here are a few essential pieces for every professional:

Necklace: Necklaces are must have in the jewelry box. They come in a variety of shapes and sizes and can be quite versatile. You can use a necklace to dress up a t-shirt or dress. Different types of necklaces include pendant necklaces, dainty, delicate necklaces, or even statement piece necklaces. For me, my everyday go-to piece of jewelry is a necklace gifted to me by my mother and goes with everything I wear. Necklaces are small but needed accessories in the closet that take little effort.

Arm Candy: Everyone loves candy, right? Bracelets are the perfect way to dress up your wrist. They come in varying shapes, sizes, metals, and colors. Bangles, cuff, and stretch bracelets can all accentuate your outfit.

Earrings: Having a pair of simple, go-to earrings is also essential. Sometimes you want to wear earrings but don't want the large hoops or dangling earrings. Studs or pearls work perfectly to give taste to any outfit. If you go with large earrings such as hoops or feathers, be sure to have a simpler outfit, so that the two do not clash. Be sure to find earrings in a color and size that make you feel comfortable enough to wear.

Rings: Always having a few rings handy can be a surefire way to add some spice to an outfit. Rings are also probably one of the easiest pieces to wear. You've got cocktail rings (big and flashy) to delicate rings (small, classic, and beautiful), which come in different styles, colors and metals. You can also opt to stack rings for an added effect. Be sure to see how they look on all of your fingers, and remember you will bring attention to your fingers, so be sure those nails are groomed.

Hats: Hats are another awesome way to accessorize outfits. They are very specific in styles, so if you are going for a preppy look or a bohemian look, adding a hat is the way to go. Even if you don't like baseball, a baseball cap is a classic to have; they can accessorize jeans and a tee. Not only do they help accessorize, but they can be a must have for bad hair days.

PART 2: STATEMENT PIECES

Statement pieces are great additions to an outfit and help take it from drab to straight fab. It is usually one piece that is bold and stands out while capturing attention. From earrings and necklaces to belts and jackets, statement pieces come in all shapes, colors and sizes. They don't have to be limited to accessories, but I have included them in this section because of the common association.

I always wear my favorite statement piece when I want my outfit to have an extra oomph feel or when I have an important meeting approaching, as it helps me feel strong, confident and feminine. Here are a few keys to statement pieces:

- Less is more: The key to making a statement piece work is to, of course, have fun, but keep it simple too. Remember, less is more. Use one eye-catching piece to bring your entire outfit together. Let the statement piece do all the talking. For example, you can throw on a pair of jeans and a white tee with a chunky silver necklace. Without the necklace, you probably wouldn't notice the outfit, but with it you certainly would.

- Necklaces: One of the most common statement pieces I see around are necklaces. These are perfect to wear with solid color dresses as they can bring so much life to the dress. It is important to match the right necklace with the right neckline. For example, necklaces look especially great with strapless or off-the-shoulder tops.

- Remember the statement piece is supposed to make a statement. It's important to wear them appropriately so that they don't make the wrong statement. If you want to give an outfit life and take it from #basic to #leveledUp, then consider adding a statement piece to your wardrobe.

PART 3: ACCESSORIES BASED ON THE OCCASION

Workplace/office: Different places of work have different rules about jewelry. Consider avoiding big and distracting pieces that may get in the way. For example, If you are using your hands often, it may not be wise to wear bangles the make loud noises every time you move your hands. Pieces such as watches (gold, silver, or even colorful ones) are smart, sophisticated and can be practical while also serving as wrist candy. Staying simple in the workplace is always a good idea.

Weekend/Date Night: It's time to take the hair down and unwind. Weekend fun (e.g. brunch with friends or date night) call for big statement pieces. Show off your bold statement necklace or your bright cocktail ring. These are the perfect settings to showcase these pieces, especially if they give you good feels!

Casual: For this setting, you want pieces that will make you feel happy, comfortable and relaxed. Consider simpler pieces like pendant necklaces, hats, or, for the winter months approaching, scarves. You should wear pieces that make you feel 100% like yourself.

Formal: Formal events include galas, balls, or official events. You want to consider pieces that may spark conversation (antique pieces, for example, as they have history behind them). You can also never go wrong with pearls or diamonds, as they give off an elegant vibe. The goal is to have classy but effortless pieces to bring your outfit together.

PART 4: BAGS

> *"Purses are like friends, you can never have too many!"*
>
> **—Unknown**

There are ways to snag a Chanel, Celine, or Gucci bag without paying full retail price. Consider purchasing a pre-owned bag from sites like Tradesy or Poshmark; often the bags are authentic and in great condition. As with jewelry, there are several types of bags to choose from:

Everyday work bag: This is the typical everyday bag that the everyday working woman NEEDS in her collection. It can help to keep you organized throughout the week with its many compartments and holders. Some work bags are versatile enough to transition into the weekend.

Oversized or roomie tote: This is the bag that is big enough to carry "it all." This is also perfect for work or when traveling to keep essentials on hand. Sometimes the totes do not have compartments, so you may want to purchase an extra compartment organizer or find a tote that is lined and has inside pockets.

The clutch: Can you say perfect for the night time or special occasion look? This is the bag for going to a party, a wedding, or out on the town for a girl's night out (GNO).

Crossbody/Sling Bag: This is the in-between bag that is perfect for the on-the-go essentials. These bags typically have a long strap that can be worn on the shoulder or across the body. This is the bag if you're out running errands or casually hanging with the crew.

PART 5: SHOES

"Give a girl the right shoes and she can conquer the world."
—Marilyn Monroe

LOOKING FOR SHOES

Shoe lovers everywhere unite! Whether you're going into the office or hanging for GNO, there is a perfect shoe for every occasion. Remember, we need our shoes to look good, but what's equally important is that they fit properly and provide adequate support. When you are searching for shoes, here are a few tips:

1. Consider trying on shoes at the end of the day. Our feet tend to swell by evening, and this will help you get your true size.

2. When trying on shoes, don't be afraid to stand and walk around in the shoes to get a good feel for them.

3. You determine if the shoes are truly comfortable, not the salesperson or the brand!

Shoes for the workplace

The number one factor when buying any type of shoe, especially for work, is the seven letter word: comfort. You want to find shoes that allow you to move around the office but still remain stylish at the same time. Finding classic colors such a black, brown, grey or nude will give you more options to match your apparel. Lastly, you want to ensure your shoes are appropriate for the company dress code.

Casual shoes

These are the shoes that you will wear on a day-to-day basis for a more relaxed look. From sneakers to flats, these shoes can fall into the casual category. Heels can also fit into the casual look, such as wedges or low heels.

GNO (Girls Night Out) shoes

Picking shoes to wear out for a night on the town can be quite the task. You want to look on point but don't want your feet hurting an hour into the evening. I feel your pain! Make sure you know the details of the evening (is it a dive bar, lounge, concert with no seating?) as this will help guide the shoes you select. As a hint, shoes with a block heel or wedges are perfect for going out.

FINAL TIPS FOR SHOES

Shoes are worth investing a little more money in because, in most cases, you get what you pay for. Investing in some classic black pumps will never go out of style and can be used for the office, a night out, or transitioned into a casual look for brunch. If you are new to heels, be sure to ease your way into them by starting small with kitten heels or wedges and slowly increasing the heel size.

Notes

Notes

Notes

Notes

Chapter 12
Appearance in the Professional Space

---◆---

"What you wear is how you present yourself to the world. Fashion is instant language."

—M. Prada

FIRST IMPRESSIONS

First impressions truly are everything: When we meet someone for the first time, there are lots of thoughts that go through our minds. We often observe how they speak, their demeanor, body language, and mannerisms, but inevitably, we often find ourselves also looking at their physical appearance. Our verbal communication skills are an important aspect of creating a great first impression, but we have to remember not to neglect the non-verbal skills too. There have been some studies that show that it takes about three seconds for someone to form an opinion about you. You want to make sure what is being conveyed about you in the first three seconds will give you a positive lasting impression because first impressions are hard to undo and often set the tone for the relationship that follows.

HYGIENE

Although it is not a highly spoken about topic, we must address it, and ladies, it's our hygiene. Personal hygiene is important because it helps to ensure good health and can also have social benefits. It can also help your self-esteem so that you feel awesome about yourself! When at work, we are around others and unpleasant odors or a shabby appearance will not want to inspire others to work with you. It can be distracting and impact your ability to perform well.

The following simple steps can help to maintain practicing daily hygiene. Washing or bathing is an important way to maintain hygiene removing dirt and odors, while protecting ourselves against possible infections and illness. The frequency of bathing or showing will vary based on individual and culture, but one should consider washing the face and body at least once every day or every other day. Hand washing should occur frequently throughout the day as this is a way to protect ourselves and others from bacteria that we may come into contact with daily.

GROOMING

For us ladies, the small details are important and count. Remember, first impressions are being made every day. Can you recall the last time you washed your hair or trimmed and cleaned your nails? How about a checkup at the dentist? Although every office environment and culture is different, there are a few basic guidelines which can be applicable everywhere:

1. No need to go full glam-on with the makeup (unless it's okay in your office setting and you want to) but wearing the few basics (mascara, concealer or foundation) can help you look awake and fresh.

2. Nails should be trimmed, clean and painted with a neutral color (again, some office environments may have different rules and allow other colors). You want to avoid overly long false nails with elaborate art.

3. As busy professionals juggling school, work, family, personal life, we can often overlook ourselves! Don't forget to schedule dental visits for cleanings to make sure you keep a pearly white smile and fresh breath.

At work, you always want your personality and best image to shine through, and not create opportunities for others to judge you. Again, hygiene will vary for some, but at the very least, your hair, nails and make-up should be appropriate.

ATTIRE

If you are new to the workplace, my biggest tip: find out the pre-requisites and dress code rules of your company. You certainly want to express yourself through fashion at work, but you want to be respectful of your company's dress code. It's also important to remember the way you dress is a direct reflection of your company. At work, we want others to focus on our professional skills, not on how we look.

Notes

Notes

Notes

Notes

Bonus:
Style on Point, How About Your Professional Skills?

Your professional style is on point. How about your professional skills?

When we look good, we feel good, and that gives us the momentum to want to achieve more. We have navigated attire for the professional space, and now it's time to make sure our skills are up to par with our style. At some point during our professional work career, we may feel stuck, want to make a career switch or level up on our skills. Sometimes learning new skills or obtaining new certifications can be pricey, but not always. In my own journey, I have gone through a few career changes that helped me learn how to gain new skills. Below are just a few ways to build up those resumes so that we can confidently go after what we want in our careers.

READING

You want to sit down and research the skills you wish to develop or learn. Google is our best friend and you can find any article or book on that topic. There is so much information available to us on the internet and often is free. If you want to become an expert in a particular field, find out who the experts are, follow them, and read their publications. Try to increase your reading every month, and I promise you will learn new information and gain new skills.

JOB SHADOWING

This is hands-on learning where you work with a person one-on-one in a field or area of expertise that you have an interest in. You are learning from someone who is doing a job that you actually want to do. Be sure to consider the skills you want to develop or improve on, whether it's public speaking or working in a lab. You can look to individuals at your current company or even at another company. If you have a friend or an acquaintance who is doing something you're interested in, reach out and ask if you can spend a few days with them. The best part about this: it's completely free and you are learning on-the-job skills.

ATTENDING CONFERENCES

This is one of my favorite ways to learn additional skills and information while also cultivating new relationships with others who have similar interests. Conference prices may vary, but some employers will cover the cost of conference attendance or reimburse some costs, as you are building on your skillset, which could be applicable to your role within the company. Simply ask. Some conferences will also provide scholarships for first-time attendees or individuals who demonstrate a financial need.

ONLINE COURSES

No matter which area of skillset you are trying to improve, you can find an online course for it. Sites such as Skillshare offer online communities where you discover or take a class in any area. Some online courses are free, and others may be less pricey. If they aren't free, I promise they are less expensive than physically attending a school. You will learn a new skill, which can be put on your resume to help you get to the next level.

Notes

Notes

Notes

Notes

Bonus:
Don't Let Your Light Burn Out

"You can't take care of anyone until you take care of you."

—Beyoncé

This is a special bonus chapter because this is a topic that professional women do not often talk about. In today's society we hear a lot about "hustling, grinding day in and day out, being a boss," but no one talk about burnout. Well burnout is very real and is something I personally dealt with in my professional career for months. We are often multi-tasking and juggling many hats such as our career, family and school! When you are burned out, there is no way to experience the glow up in your life. I'm here to let you know that burnout, especially for us professional women, can happen and is important for us to recognize if it occurs and how to deal with it.

What is burnout? According to Webster's Dictionary, it's "the physical or mental collapse caused by overwork or stress." My interactions with my colleagues at work changed and this even trickled over into my personal life and interaction with friends and family. At the time, I didn't identify it as such, because I thought "this is what everyone who is grinding goes through." I was sleeping more, had no energy, and always felt stressed out. My attitude toward going to work changed. I was no longer excited about my job, my interactions with my patients and those I worked with changed. I did not have the energy to be productive at work, had difficulty concentrating, and just did not feel satisfied with my job. I simply felt overwhelmed.

Why is it important that we address this state of burnout? It certainly impacts our mental, physical and emotional health, which affects our performance at work. Burnout can also increase our risk for certain diseases such as depression, diabetes, hypertension, heart disease and fatigue. I shared what I experience, but burnout can present in many different ways. A few symptoms to be aware of include:

- Feeling extremely exhausted, no matter how much rest you get
- Feeling overwhelmed
- Not feeling satisfied with your accomplishments at work
- Easily irritable with others
- You have no control over your workload

When burnout occurs, it does not mean you've done anything wrong or that you need to quit your job. It simply means you need to re-evaluate your situation, first understanding why this is happening. For myself, I was trying to do too much at one time and not prioritizing one thing: me. So if you believe you are experiencing burnout, take a step back and look at the overall picture at home or at work. Ask yourself what is going on to make me feel this way and reflect on how you reached this space. Once we understand the why, we can try to make the appropriate changes to reverse burnout.

It is also important to reach out and seek support. I began reaching out to my mentors and loved ones for support. I learned that I was not the only one and others wanted to help me. I also spoke to my supervisor to see what changes could be implemented to help relieve some of the responsibilities at work. Although it can be challenging, consider incorporating small amounts of physical activity (such as walking or yoga) into your routine. These types of activities can serve as an outlet for stress and take our mind off work. Lastly, we must cut ourselves some slack. We simply cannot be everything to everyone, and we have to prioritize ourselves at the end of the day. Remember, if you are not feeling well and not in a good space, you will not be any good to anyone.

Notes

Notes

Notes

Notes

Thank You

---◆---

I want to thank you for purchasing this book and taking the time to read it. I hope that you found it useful to help build your confidence, and create your professional style so that you can achieve your goals, as these are a few of the tips that have helped me. I also want to thank all the beautiful women whose actions helped mold me into the lady I am today. I am extremely grateful and thankful to God, because without him I would not be here. To my future husband Helal, thank you for being my die hard supporter and encouraging me to take leaps. To my mother Rose, who showed me what it means to be a resilient woman. Thankful to my father Herb, who taught me the importance of hard work. Grateful to my stepdad Phil, who treated and loved me as his own. Thankful to my beautiful sister Jamie, who is always an incredible shoulder to lean on. A huge thank you to my brother Lamar, who inspired me to pursue medicine and taught me never to take the small things in life for granted. A very special shout out and thank you to my coach Dr. Toni, who pushed me beyond my comfort zone.

About the Author

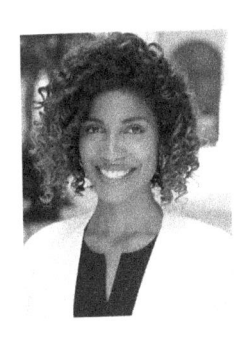

Leveraging her professional background in medicine paired with a natural flair for beauty and style, Dr. Kristamarie Collman takes a holistic approach in helping professional women to enhance their lives. She offers tips and advice on a range of topics including healthy eating, professional style, and beauty hacks.

Dr. Kristamarie earned her medical degree from New York Medical College and joined the ranks of Halifax Health Medical Center as a resident physician shortly after graduation. Named as Chief Resident 2015–2016, Dr. Kristamarie serves as a family medicine physician specializing in lifestyle medicine, weight management, and nutrition.

Dr. Kristamarie is also a social media influencer that has captured the hearts of thousands around the country. She is the co-founder of Young Ladies Watching, a nonprofit organization empowering underrepresented women pursuing healthcare related careers.

Dr. Kristamarie practices her wellness messages through running, cooking, and spending time with her husband and two dogs.

To connect, visit her website at www.drkristamarie.com

purposely created
PUBLISHING

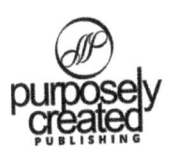

CREATING DISTINCTIVE BOOKS
WITH INTENTIONAL RESULTS

We're a collaborative group of creative masterminds with a mission to produce high-quality books to position you for monumental success in the marketplace.

Our professional team of writers, editors, designers, and marketing strategists work closely together to ensure that every detail of your book is a clear representation of the message in your writing.

Want to know more?
Write to us at info@publishyourgift.com
or call (888) 949-6228

Discover great books, exclusive offers, and more at
www.PublishYourGift.com

Connect with us on social media

@publishyourgift